7 DAYS TO A HEALTHY

LIFESTYLE

Larry A. Cochran, MBA

7 DAYS TO A HEALTHY LIFESTYLE

ISBN: 978-0-557-20416-8

Table of Content

Acknowledgements

Dedicated to My Wife Angela

who is on this journey toward good health with me

and

To coach Wallace

who sparked the love for knowing my body back in high school

Preface

This book comes along at a time that I am looking to revamp my entire life. It is set in a time of great comfort knowing that life is a gift and we have to do all that we can to live healthy and well. As a believer in Christ, most people believe that this issue is only one that can be dealt with on the secular side, but this is where they would be wrong. Although I am going to deal with this on a basic issue for the sake of keeping the text clear and short, I want to keep everyone fully persuaded in my biblical stance. Life is a gift from God and we must not waste it. We should preserve all times under the grace that He has provided us. This book is a declaration to all who have decided to take a real stance. It is not exhaustive, but rather a stepping stone toward the life of health and wellness that no one is guaranteed to have outside of hard work and dedication to it. Good luck on your journey. Be well and of good cheer, grace is with you all.

Forward

TO BE ADDED IN REPRINT

Introduction

My life has taken many turns, some for the better and some for the worst. As a youth I was said to have all the athletic ability in the world, with the potential to go professional one day, if life plays itself out in the right way. I was in great shape all throughout my youth and young adult life. Playing sports in high school and then in college, I was sure that my lifestyle was one of good health and longevity. I had never suffered any of the ailments that were hereditary for my family and life seemed to be going well. Why write a book about health and lifestyle? Well, I am not that teenager with all the potential in the world. I am the average adult with declining physical stamina, a heavy workload, a busy schedule, diminishing eyesight, and a host of other ailments. I am just the average guy. Life does not have to end because the dream of eternal youth has somehow come to heads with reality. I am an average guy with an average ability with an average lifestyle. This is why I have set on the journey to simplify the results that I once thought was only in my youth. We can have a greater health and wellness lifestyle than we did when we were younger. The reality is that when we were younger we had biology and chemistry on our side, when we grow older; these very same things seem to work against us. Or do they?

There are some very simple steps that we can take to have a much better life, a more sustainable physical appearance, a strong self-awareness, and longer life overall. Starting with the decision to make the change, you have placed yourself on the right path. Yet being on the right path does not guarantee that you will get anywhere, you must have a road map for where you are or where you want to be. Knowing yourself is essential to the process, but without a realistic stance on humility, you will only be spinning your wheels and end up following trend after trend or fad after fad. This is not a healthy lifestyle to pursue. I recommend through the chapters things like: changing what you say about dieting and exercise, changing what and how you eat, and finally changing what you do to sustain your healthy lifestyle. This booklet is a guideline that can be drawn upon from time to time to give you a quick jumpstart back into the world of health and wellness. Take as long as you need to get through each day, as to each day may not actually last 24 hours but a week or even longer, depending on your ability to adapt the tasks and carry them through. Be strong and courageous as you start this journey toward a healthy lifestyle.

Author and fitness guru, John Basedow, has made it his mission to give people hope in reaching fitness goals. His mantra, which he constantly repeats is "What you are today doesn't necessarily indicate what you'll be tomorrow" (Basedow, 2008).

Where to start

GETTING DOWN TO

BUSINESS

Day 1 – Make the decision to stop dieting

This chapter deals with the problem of having a dieting mentality. Dieting is about losing unwanted weight that has been gain and does not always equate to lifestyle changes. Dieting leads to more dieting, while lifestyle changes lead to less reliance on dieting. What works with dieting? What does not work with dieting? Why go for lifestyle change rather than ordinary dieting? Dieting is trendy and all about the current fad.

Its no big secret that fad dieting doesn't work for the typical American. The only problem is that most diet plans that have come out in recent years are not based on good science. The American Dietetic Association, Dieticians of Canada, and American College of Sports Medicine all claim that there must be a proper distribution of nutritional needs met for every individuals (Journal of American Diet Association, 2000). The United States Department of Agriculture understands that one size does not fit all[1], yet this seems to be the contrary statement made by most fad diet inventors. Fad diets make very sensational claims. These claims will offer recommendations that offer a quick fix, recommendations on studies that ignore differences in individuals or groups, dramatic statements that are refuted by reputable scientific organizations, or recommendations made to help sell a product[2]. When looking to overhaul your physical, nutritional, spiritual, or mental health it is vital to understand that a change in the habits that led to the current problems has to be taken into consideration. On day two, we will evaluate what may have caused some of the problems in your diet and nutritional life. Today we want to look at and understand the difference between a fad diet and a real diet. We want to explore the notion of regular dieting activities and an overall lifestyle lift.

> By definition, a lifestyle is a characteristic bundle
>
> of behaviors that makes sense to both others

---

[1] United States Department of Agriculture (USDA) – http://www.mypyramid.gov

[2] WebMD – (Website maintained by doctors under scrutiny of a medical review board) – http://www.webmd.com

and oneself in a given time and place, including social relations, consumption, entertainment, and dress. The behaviors and practices within lifestyles are a mixture of habits, conventional ways of doing things, and reasoned actions. A lifestyle typically also reflects an individual's attitudes, values or worldview. Therefore, a lifestyle is a means of forging a sense of self and to create cultural symbols that resonate with personal identity. Not all aspects of a lifestyle are entirely voluntary. Surrounding social and technical systems can constrain the lifestyle choices available to the individual and the symbols she/he is able to project to others and the self[3].

To change a lifestyle requires time and dedication. The fact that you are now reading this book tells me that you probably

---

[3] Wikipedia – (Free online encyclopedia) - http://en.wikipedia.org/wiki/Lifestyle#cite_note-1

believe that you don't have either. You have to make the choice to stop the merry-go-round of dieting and exercise fads. There has to be an unwavering attitude toward good health and nutrition. Habits are not too quickly broken. They are stubborn and hard to break away from. Since we have no time to spare, let us get to the purpose of this booklet, the task of the day.

DAY ONE TASK

The task for today is to begin with the choice to eat right, exercise right, and live right. Without this commitment, the rest of this book will be useless to you. Stay focused on the task at hand. Be ready to move from simply thinking about what you want to do about your health to actually doing something tangible about your health. So that this day will be available to be built upon, I will have you do a few things. Number one; go grab a pen and some paper. Number two; write down the exact goals that you have in mind for your health and wellness. We will work through them together to help you achieve these goals. Remember that they must be realistic and very much attainable. Make sure that they are not so easy that they leave no room for ambition. The goals that you have on paper now will be refined as you go through this booklet. The main idea of this text is not to give a quick fix, but rather to put you on the road to recovery.

Day 2 – Know thyself

What are some of the reasons that have lead to the lifestyle that you have today? How was your family life as it pertains to health and wellness? How has your relationships shaped your health and wellness? How is your schedule shaping your lifestyle? In order to move into a healthy lifestyle, you need to know how you arrived at the point you are today? There is a role that socioeconomic factors and socio-political context has in determining health related lifestyles that is seldom referenced (Korp, 2008; Cokerham, 2005).

As I have recently begun to understand is that we know very little about anything or any given subject, but there is one subject that we should all be well-informed about, that is ourselves. To know yourself is to have more than a series of surface facts about those things that you are consciously aware of and believe that you can control or change, but you need to be armed with the information about yourself that you may only subconsciously aware of and my not be able to change. That is, you can not change without help from someone or something outside yourself. I am sure that you did not intently fall on the beaten path of improper and unhealthy life choices, but rather it was a slowly enticing life of giving in to certain deep urges until one day you suddenly awoke and asked yourself, how this could have possibly occurred. If you are one of the few people who have been brought up by right thinkers in the area of health and wellness, great for you, but if you are one of the countless others who were victims of internal and external factors that contributed to your current behavior, this is for you.

As we alluded to on the previous day, habits are hard to break. Even so, habits are not as hard to form. One thing that we must overcome to have a better healthy lifestyle is our environment. For instance, people who live in low-income neighborhoods have issues to overcome such an abundance of convenient stores that sell things like tobacco and alcohol, but lack fresh markets that sell items like fresh fruits and vegetables (Docksai, 2009). Continued efforts are being thrust out aimed at these communities to help increase awareness about the potential risk factors about drugs and alcohol, but these alone are not enough? There has to be a change in the total environment. There was a research done to say that environment plays very little on eating habits (Hackett et al, 2008). This study only dealt with the issue of desert as a food choice. It did not bring to mind the entire environment that influences choice. To fully grasp the influence of our environment, we have to include all factors involved in that environment.

Today more than ever we are products of overwork as well as overeating as well as under sleeping. We spend more time doing and less time recharging from doing. We spend more time moving forward physically than we do refueling the body with the proper nutrients needed to survive another day of grueling events. Our lives have become filled with friends and habits that push us to our limits, but refuse to allow us the opportunity to recoup. We need an environment that will be calming and relaxing. Habitus expresses the idea that people make choices, but their choices are always constrained and influenced by resources and social identity (Korp, 2008). We need an open schedule from time to time to do nothing. When our schedule is packed, it brings to our rescue the worst medicine we could have ever called for, fast foods. The major issue with fast food in our hectic schedule is not convenience because it is available everywhere, all the time, and now for very little. The problem with fast food is that it is loaded with things our bodies need little or none of at all. We look at our food labels and say we know what we are putting in, but that is only half the battle. Let say you have a cheeseburger, just and average one, not an Angus. That cheeseburger has 24% of your dietary fat, 35% saturated; it has 26% of your dietary cholesterol, 63% of your dietary protein. This is just the burger. This burger has 480 calories toward an average 2000 calorie diet[4]. Your nutritional day has not much more room for error after this. We have not added fries or drinks to the equation. Some people even have two burgers, God forbid. You can see where this one is headed.

---

[4] Fit Day – (Website created to help count daily caloric intake) - http://www.fitday.com/WebFit/nutrition/All_Foods/Meat_Beef_Pork_Misc_/Cheeseburger_1_4_lb_meat_beef_modified_in_fat_content_with_tomato_and_or_catsup_on_bun.html

Our food choices are just the tip of the iceberg when it comes to dealing with diet and exercise habits. Our environment and the issues that it brings to us is another factor.

DAY TWO TASK

Today, we are going to have you explore some of your personal daily habits by keeping a dietary log. The log should begin with the time you went to sleep the night before and end when you lay down to sleep on the next day. There has to be a full twenty-four hour cycle recorded. There is a resource in the back of this booklet in the resource section (p???) that will help you on this journey. Do not cheat. We will be discussing a few other items within this day of recording in order to accurately your habits. Repeat this for a minimum of 3 days in order to kill the notion that this is just a one time thing. Own the day; own the idea of personal responsibility. Take the time to do this accurately and properly. When you come back in later days to review these logs, you will see what habits you may not even know that you have obtained over time. In the log, we will account for your environment. Answer the questionnaire before starting your log and this will help to trace some of the heretical traits behind the habits as well.

Knowing is just the beginning

ACTIONS

Day 3 – What are you saying?

Things that we say to ourselves will affect how we approach all subjects, including health and wellness. Speaking negatively is only one part of what we say to ourselves that will hinder our efforts to diet and exercise. There are other words that are less suspecting, but carry the same weight. Telling yourself that you are losing weight for any reason other than for health is a recipe for disaster. Health and wellness begins with the right self talk, it begins with positive affirmations, strategic planning, and strong dedication.

We have already worked on finding our patterns, and understanding our motivations from the outside of ourselves. Now is the time to deal with the inner voices of unreason. We have a tendency to down talk ourselves in ways that we don't even realize. We are all familiar with terms such as I can't do that, this will never work, or I don't have the discipline to follow through. These are some of the ways in which we speak negatively against our progress, but they are only a small portion of the negative talk that we experience from ourselves. The talking down our own ability to complete any task starts much prior to the time when we decide to take on that task. This paralyzing speech may even sound encouraging at the time prior because we have not even begun taking on the life style change to this level. Here are some of those sayings that may pop up prior to even thinking of making this type of lifestyle change:

"Exercise really doesn't have a benefit"

"Eating right is not really relevant"

"I am contented with my life in every way and won't need to change much"

These phrase are harmless we think if we are in the context of our youth, or when we are confident that we are not going in the wrong direction. This is why they are not thought of as a problem prior to your decision to make a lifestyle change. These ideas come long before there is a diagnosis of a problem. The reality is that you did not take the idea that bad health and poor lifestyle could ever be your problem. That actually started your problem. No one is immune to a poor lifestyle or bad and negative health. While some things are environmental, others have risks that can be significantly reduced even before the onset of any problem. The only dilemma that we are all faced with is dealing with those demons that come to haunt us over inner statements and some verbal statements that we have made at some time in the past, prior to us realizing that we may have a problem. Another area in this type of negative self-talk is saying things that may send your goals off into the wrong direction.

This other area of negative self-talk deals with the actual words we use to excuse ourselves from doing what we know is needful for enhanced life enjoyment or just for plain health reasons. If you tell yourself that you are losing weight to fit into a dress, or that you are going to stop drinking alcohol because of what it does to others and how they see you, these are not very strong or sustaining reasons. As a matter of fact they are both temporal and can cause very serious fallbacks in the long run. What happens after you have fit that dress? What happens if that person you became sober for walks out? These are seriously designed approaches for relapse. The real reason for all lifestyle changes is personal and health related. To some degree, everything that we do and say will affect and have some effect on our overall health. To keep smoking when you are fully aware that lung cancer is a strong possibility, while on the other hand saying that you want to life long and have a healthy life are opposing ideas. To say that smoking at a young and energetic time in your life will not affect your overall health later is just plain silly. Scientific evidence shows that keeping a positive outlook helps us to stay healthy and live longer (Small, 2006).

DAY THREE TASK

Today is a simple day. All that is going to be done is to make a valiant attempt to repent from all of the negative ideas, talk, and thoughts that may have contributed to the lifestyle that you are living today. We want to fully accept our part in our current reality. Without accepting full credit for what you have done or said to yourself, that may have contributed to the lifestyle that you now live, is going to hinder your ability to take future actions. Ultimately, you are the one responsible for where you are today, both negatively and positively. If you have congratulated yourself for your accomplishments in the past, today you must repent for you failure to guard your own heart against the things that are now plaguing your life. Today, repent or turn from those early ideas that are not productive to your good health and well-ness.

Day 4 – What am I eating?

No healthy lifestyle is sustainable without the proper diet and nutrition. What we put into our bodies is equally as important as what we do to our bodies. Our physical mobility, physical stamina, and even our psychological capabilities can be impaired by bad nutritional habits. The human body has biological needs that can be met through the intake of certain foods and beverages. In order to decide what foods we need, we must all investigate the various aspects of our individual make up. Those areas can include but are not limited to: blood type, personal physical demands, body type, personal taste, environmental factors, and heredity factors. After looking at our own limitations, we must learn how to read labels and how these items that we will intake will affect us emotionally, physically, biologically, and intellectually.

As we discussed in day two, there has to be a clear understanding of how the environment may have impacted your overall health. If you are forced to remain living in an area that does not have the kind of fresh food markets that another community may have, you are going to have to make a decision to not allow that to hinder what you will need to do. The things that we put into our body are so detrimental to our health that we need to be fully aware of what those things are. Money should never be the thing that stops good eating habits, since the greater cost in actually poor health in the long term. Eating less of a good thing is better than an abundance of bad foods. We have to get out of the habit of living to eat, but rather knowing how to eat to live. When a person lives their lives around certain planned eating requirements that can be dangerous, but equally so is the idea of eating poorly and ignorantly. There is a right way and a wrong way to eat. In the task that will follow, we will give one example of the right way. Learning how to eat is going to be some thing that is a great benefit.

DAY FOUR TASK

To get to the point, there are few ideas that must be understood tradition has been lost. Industrial foods are the opposite of real foods (Planck, 2006). Industrial food is more synthetic today and is really only intended to be a replica of what was once traditional.

Eating the right types of food is one part of that change in our eating lifestyle. Next, we need to know how to eat these things. There are three major meals and three optional snack times that we have each day. For the sake of brevity here is the basic rule of thumb, breakfast should be the largest meal, since your body has a great amount of time to digest and use the nutrients. Lunch should be modest, yet filling. Dinner should be the lightest meal of the day and should be taken at least 2 to 3 hours before going to bed. In order to not go to bed hungry, add a snack after dinner about and hour after. Also for health reasons, please remember to brush before bed. We are talking about brushing because whether we want to admit it or not, some of the toothpaste is dietary, but so is that food that may remain on your teeth rotting over night. Let's kill two birds with one stone, let's get rid of the rotting food, and let's put down that hunger bug. Today, eat, and eat right.

Finally, read the labels of the foods that you are ingesting. Do not eat anything that you have not understood the ingredients that are included in that item. Go to the government website that actually trains you on how to read labels[5]. Yeah, there is a website that trains you for free how to read labels. There are also interactive trainings available to those who like presentations and computer training modules. Also, learn how to make your calories a more affective part of your eating[6].

---

[5] FDA-
http://www.fda.gov/Food/LabelingNutrition/ConsumerInformation/ucm078889.htm
[6] FDA -
http://www.fda.gov/Food/LabelingNutrition/ConsumerInformation/ucm114022.htm

Day 5 – What am I doing?

After knowing where you are and where you have come from, along with what habits you may have, it is now time to understand where you are physically. The actions that are taken today must reflect the desired outcome required. Whether the preference is to expand on current capabilities or just to improve them, a healthy lifestyle is one of the primary tasks needed. Thinking things through from the beginning can be a valuable step; yet taking action is the ultimate goal in the equation of health and wellness. Ask yourself, what am I doing and what should I be doing? Then project actions by asking what will I do now? What are the needful steps that will change the current circumstances from bad to good or from good to great?

Fix your brain for longevity and your body will follow in kind (Small, 2006). By keeping our minds sharp, we are more inclined to stay physically fit. As stated previously, scientific evidence shows that keeping a positive outlook helps us to stay healthy and live longer. Small states that the 8 essential tips for longevity include: sharpening your mind, keeping a positive outlook, cultivating healthy and intimate relationships, promoting stress-free living, staying in shape, and using modern medicine (Small, 2006).

Because our environment has a very direct impact on how we feel, it is important to make sure that the environment is functional. Keeping our lives clutter free is a great way to maintain a functioning environment. This issue of clutter free living is further expanded in the booklet, *7 Days to a clutter free life*, which will be hitting the press soon. When creating a comfortable home or work environment it is essential to place the focus on function (Small, 2006), you may also want to deal with the emotional impact of the space (Small, 2006). One example is that of having too many decorations, which can be uninviting and uncomfortable to even the person who owns that home or office.

Dealing with the issue of exercise is not as simple, but not very complex in terms of the availability of programs out there. First we all must understand that there is no shame in trying out different programs of fitness. The primary premise has been overwhelmingly accepted to be that not all programs are alike and not all programs work for everyone. Being able to choose a program that is right for you is an advantage in today's era of modern medicine and modern technology. This is a sad day when technology and medicine has advanced, but our overall health and wellness seems to be declining. What is the missing component? Personal responsibility is the missing component. Science is teaching us that we have many differences that are so subtle that we would benefit most from specialized programs for exercise, diet, nutrition, and other health related areas. When we take responsibility, we see the need to be concerned for our health. A good fitness routine for exercise will cover cardiovascular conditioning, balance and flexibility, and strength training (Small, 2006). Make sure you know your maximum heart rate, which is calculated by subtracting your age from 220. The actual heart rate, when engaging in exercise, should remain between 70 to 90% of the maximum heart rate for maximum impact.

Great cardiovascular exercise to use in some kind of rotational mix are things like walking, jogging, swimming, cycling, sports, dancing, aerobics, housework, and gardening. Some flexibility and balance ideas are Tai Chi, Yoga, stretching, and stability balls. Finally, for weight training, consider weight machines, free weights, and resistance bands (Small, 2006).

DAY FIVE TASK

Today's task is very simple. Start exercising. Start with something very light like walking for 30 minutes. As you begin to work out a routine pattern, then you can become more creative. The first step in this healthy lifestyle has to begin with starting a good habit. When the day is done, make sure that you have begun to exercise, remembering each of the three components: cardiovascular, balance and flexibility, and strength training. Have fun also. One way to jumpstart a healthy lifestyle program is by visiting an exercise or fitness fair. Participating in events such as "Healthy living made fun", which is a day long event promoting a healthy lifestyle, is a great spark for the fire. Taking part in these types of events can help inform you as well as inspire you.

"it is great to see people exercising and pampering themselves" quote from a volunteer helper, Liz Grundy (Gibbons & Pointu, 2009).

Getting to the heart of the matter

WRAPPING UP

Day 6 – Who is supporting me?

In the book "The 100 Year Lifestyle", Dr. Eric Plasker speaks about surrounding yourself with a circle of influence. He lists seven things to do to bring companionship into your life. There is a mention of things like eating with a friend, going for a walk, going to the gym, going shopping, going on vacations, or being devoted to a cause. I would like to add attend a local church gathering or bible study group. This booklet has dealt specifically with the healthy lifestyle portion which would be directly associated with things like going to the gym, going for a walk, and eating. Having some one to workout with can make it less daunting and in some cases even fun. Our habits can also be either encouraged or discouraged by the people that we are continually around and associate with. What kind of support base do you have? Dr. Plasker suggest that you start a support group with yourself (Plasker, 2007)

As stated in the previous day's evaluation, a very important to have the right relationships when attempting to make any life

51

changes. The people that are around you can help to make or break your momentum in the process. When family and close friends are not readily available there are options for joining fitness or diet clubs (Costain & Croker, 2005). Group fitness has the benefit of setting an obligation to meet with someone, which is more likely to be followed through. While this does not always work, it can be helpful with looking to build a habit in fitness. Family members can also play a role in helping individuals form this habit, if they are involved with the fitness process as well, but the danger comes when they quit.

DAY SIX TASK

All we need today is to begin evaluating our relationships. Start thinking closely about those people who are givers in your relationship and those that are takers in your relationships; There has to be a mutual relationship that exists in your relationships. If you are the constant giver and this is draining you, stop it. People can drain more than just your finances. Think of areas to manage such as time drainers, attitude drainers, and energy drainers.

Make sure that you are nurturing the relationships that are nurturing you.

Day 7 – Forming a lasting habit

Starting strong is only part of the healthy lifestyle equation. It would be a waste of time to start strong only to drop off a week or even a month later. That is dieting and not a lifestyle. That is also a fad or trend and not a habit. Since we are calling this a lifestyle change means that we are calling for overhauls in thinking and actions, which will lead to changes in daily habits. We are all creatures of habit. We have habits that are good and then we have habits that are bad. Therefore, those habits must be geared toward a healthy lifestyle.

DAY SEVEN TASK

Start today by reviewing the previous 6 days. End today by doing days 3 through 4 continually. Knowing what you should say, knowing what you should eat, and knowing what you should do are vital to the continuation of a good healthy lifestyle.

RESOURCES

United States Department of Agriculture (USDA) –

http://www.mypyramid.gov

WebMD – (Website maintained by doctors under scrutiny of a

medical review board) – http://www.webmd.com

NOTES & BIBLIOGRAPHY

Unknown Author (2000) Position of the American Dietetic
   Association, Dieticians of Canada, and the American College
   of Sports Medicine: Nutrition and athletic performance,
   Journal of American Dietetic Association, Volume 100, Issue
   12, p. 1543-56

Docksai, R (May/June 2009) Healthy people need healthy
      communities, The Futurist, Volume 43, Issue 3, p.10,
      Published by World Future Society

Hackett, A; Boddy, L; Boothby, J; Dummer, T J; Johnson, B,
      Stratton, G (October 2008) Mapping dietary habits may
      provide clues about the factors that determine food
      choice, Journal of Nutrition and Dietetics, Volume 21,
      Issue 5, p.427-438

Basedow, J (2008) Fitness made simple, McGraw-Hill Publishing,
      New York, NY, 1st Edition, 276 Pages

Korp, P (June 2008) The symbolic power of 'health lifestyles',
      Healthy Sociology Review, Volume 17, Issue 1 p. 18-
      26, E-Content Management Pty Ltd

Planck, N (2006) real food: what to eat and why, first edition,
Bloomsbury Publishing company, New York, NY

Small, G (2006) The longevity bible: 8 essential strategies for
keeping your mind sharp and your body young,
Hyperion Publishing, New York, NY, 1st edition

Gibbons, S; Pointu, A (October 2009) Healthy living made fun,
Learning disability practice, volume 12, number 8, p.22,
RCN Publishing Company

Costain, L; Croker, H (2005) Helping individuals to help
themselves, Proceedings from the Nutrition Society,
Volume 64, p. 89-96, Cambridge University Press

Other Completed Works by this Author:

7 Days to a Healthy Lifestyle

7 Days of Time Management Planning

7 Day Series Compilation

Books and Manuscripts in the Works by this Author:

Realizing My Dreams Regardless of my Father

Misguided "The Black Identity Crisis in America"

Children's Series

"Fly Darice Fly"

Author Contact Information:

Larry A. Cochran, MBA

7335 S. Woodward Ave. Apt 212

Woodridge, IL. 60517

Phone: (708) 829-7847

Email: skollarrock@yahoo.com

Website: http://larrycochran.webs.com/

Blog: http://trufound.blogspot.com

www.ingramcontent.com/pod-product-compliance
Lightning Source LLC
Chambersburg PA
CBHW070326290526
45791CB00003B/1274